Fit and Focused: Health and Fitness for Young Professionals

Rizwan Raheem Ahmed, Ph.D.

DEDICATION

This book is dedicated to my Late Mother and Father who have provided me the financial, emotional, and Parental opportunities to raise me, provided higher education and supported me in my initial professional life journey.

TABLE OF CONTENTS

ACKNOWLEDGMENTS

I Acknowledge my wife who has supported me during writing this book. She has also helped me to generate book cover and other relevant material on Photoshop. She has encouraged me all the way in my journey.

INTRODUCTION

Health and Fitness in the Modern World

In today's fast-paced world, it can be challenging to maintain a healthy and active lifestyle. With busy work schedules and the constant pressure to meet deadlines, many young professionals find it difficult to prioritize their health and fitness. However, the benefits of leading a healthy lifestyle cannot be overstated. Regular exercise and a balanced diet can help you feel better, look better, and perform better at work. In this chapter, we will explore some of the most effective ways to stay fit and healthy in the modern world.

Weight Loss for Busy Professionals

Losing weight can be a challenge for anyone, but it can be especially difficult for busy professionals who don't have much time to dedicate to exercise and meal planning. However, there are several strategies that can help you achieve your weight loss goals without sacrificing your work or social life. These include incorporating more physical activity into your daily routine, making healthy food choices, and finding ways to reduce stress and improve sleep.

Yoga for Stress Relief and Relaxation

Yoga is a great way to de-stress and relax after a busy day at work. It can help you improve your flexibility, balance, and posture, as well as reduce anxiety and promote feelings of calmness and relaxation. Whether you prefer to practice yoga at a studio or in the comfort of your own home, there are plenty of resources available to help you get started.

CrossFit for Beginners

CrossFit is a high-intensity workout program that combines strength training, cardio, and gymnastics. It can be a great way to challenge yourself physically and mentally, but it's important to approach it with caution if you're a beginner. Make sure to start slowly and gradually increase the intensity of your workouts over time.

Paleo Diet for Athletes

The Paleo diet is a popular eating plan that emphasizes whole, unprocessed foods and excludes grains, dairy, and processed foods. It has been touted as a great option for athletes who want to improve their performance and recover more quickly from workouts. However, it's important to make sure you're getting enough nutrients and calories to support your activity level.

Running for Weight Loss

Running is a great way to burn calories and lose weight, but it's important to approach it safely and gradually. Make sure to start with a manageable distance and pace, and gradually increase both as your fitness improves. Additionally, make sure to invest in a good pair of running shoes to prevent injury and discomfort.

Senior Fitness and Mobility

Staying active and mobile becomes even more important as we age. Regular exercise can help improve balance, flexibility, and overall health in seniors, helping to maintain independence and quality of life. There are plenty of programs and resources available to help seniors stay active, including senior fitness classes and low-impact workouts.

Plant-Based Nutrition for Improved Health

A plant-based diet can be a great option for anyone looking to improve their health and reduce their risk of chronic diseases. It emphasizes whole, unprocessed foods such as fruits, vegetables, whole grains, and legumes, and excludes animal products. However, it's important to make sure you're getting enough protein, vitamins, and minerals from plant-based sources.

High-Intensity Interval Training (HIIT) for Fat Loss

HIIT is a popular workout style that combines short bursts of high-intensity exercise with periods of rest or low-intensity exercise. It can be a great way to burn calories and lose fat, but it's important to approach it with care, as it can be very intense. Make sure to start slowly and gradually increase the intensity of your workouts over time.

Strength Training for Women

Strength training is a great way to build muscle, improve bone density, and boost metabolism. Contrary to popular belief, it's also a great option for women, and can help improve overall health and fitness. Make sure to start with light weights and gradually increase the resistance over time.

Mindful Meditation for Mental and Physical Wellness

Meditation is a great way to reduce stress and improve mental and physical wellness. It can help you improve focus, reduce anxiety, and promote feelings of calmness and relaxation. There are many resources available to help you get started with meditation, including guided meditations, apps, and classes.

In conclusion, living a healthy and active lifestyle is essential for young professionals looking to succeed in their personal and professional lives. Whether you prefer yoga, CrossFit, running, or strength training, there are many options available to help you achieve your fitness goals. Additionally, making healthy food choices and finding ways to reduce stress and improve sleep can help you feel better and perform better at work. By prioritizing your health and fitness, you can achieve success in all areas of your life.

The Importance of Health and Fitness for Young Professionals

As young professionals, it can be challenging to find the time and energy to prioritize our health and fitness. With demanding work schedules, social commitments, and personal responsibilities, it's easy to neglect our physical and mental well-being. However, making health and fitness a priority is crucial for our long-term success and happiness.

Maintaining a healthy lifestyle can help us manage stress, improve our energy levels, and increase our productivity. Exercise releases endorphins, which can reduce feelings of anxiety and depression, and boost our mood. Regular physical activity also helps us sleep better, which is essential for our overall health and well-being.

In addition to the mental benefits, exercise can also improve our physical health. It can reduce the risk of chronic diseases such as heart disease, diabetes, and obesity. A healthy diet is also crucial for maintaining good health. Consuming a balanced diet with plenty of fruits, vegetables, lean proteins, and whole grains can provide us with the nutrients we need to thrive.

There are many different forms of exercise and nutrition plans to suit our individual needs and preferences. Yoga is an excellent option for stress relief and relaxation, while CrossFit can be a great way to challenge ourselves and build strength. The Paleo diet is popular among athletes, while plant-based nutrition can improve our overall health.

High-intensity interval training (HIIT) is an effective way to burn fat and increase our fitness levels in a short amount of time, while strength training can help women build lean muscle mass and boost their metabolism. Mindful meditation is a powerful tool for improving our mental and physical wellness.

It's never too late to start prioritizing our health and fitness, regardless of our age or fitness level. By making small changes to our lifestyle, such as incorporating regular exercise and eating a balanced diet, we can improve our overall health and well-being. Remember, taking care of ourselves is not a luxury, but a necessity for living a happy and fulfilling life.

The Outline of the Book

The outline of the book "Fit and Focused: Health and Fitness for Young Professionals" is designed to help young female and male professionals achieve their health and fitness goals despite their busy schedules. The book is divided into twelve chapters, each focused on specific topics that cater to different niches including health and fitness, weight loss for busy professionals, yoga for stress relief and relaxation, CrossFit for beginners, paleo diet for athletes, running for weight loss, senior fitness and mobility, plant-based nutrition for improved health, high-intensity interval training (HIIT) for fat loss, strength training for women, and mindful meditation for mental and physical wellness.

Chapter one introduces the importance of maintaining a healthy lifestyle for young professionals and provides an overview of the book. Chapter two focuses on nutrition and includes information on healthy eating habits, food groups, and portion control. Chapter three is all about exercise and the benefits it has for the body. The chapter highlights different types of exercises and recommends workout routines for different niches.

Chapter four is dedicated to weight loss for busy professionals and provides practical tips on how to lose weight without compromising work productivity. Chapter five introduces yoga as a form of exercise and relaxation. The chapter details different yoga poses, techniques, and benefits.

Chapter six discusses CrossFit, a high-intensity workout that combines weightlifting, cardio, and gymnastics. The chapter provides tips for beginners and emphasizes the importance of proper form and technique to avoid injury. Chapter seven delves into the paleo diet, a diet that focuses on consuming whole, unprocessed foods.

Chapter eight is all about running and how it can aid in weight loss. The chapter provides tips for beginners and recommends running routines for different fitness levels. Chapter nine focuses on senior fitness and mobility, providing information on exercises that can aid in maintaining mobility and preventing injuries.

Chapter ten introduces plant-based nutrition and how it can improve overall health. The chapter provides information on plant-based food sources and how to incorporate them into daily meals. Chapter eleven discusses high-intensity interval training (HIIT) as an effective form of exercise for fat loss. The chapter provides a HIIT workout routine for beginners.

Chapter twelve is dedicated to strength training for women. The chapter provides tips on how to build muscle and tone the body through weightlifting exercises. Finally, the book concludes with a chapter on mindful meditation, emphasizing the importance of mental and physical wellness and providing techniques for relaxation and stress relief.

Overall, "Fit and Focused: Health and Fitness for Young Professionals" provides a comprehensive guide to help young professionals achieve their health and fitness goals despite their busy schedules. The book caters to different niches and provides practical tips and recommendations for each. It is a must-read for anyone looking to improve their health and fitness in a sustainable way.

CHAPTER 1: HEALTH AND FITNESS BASICS

Understanding the Basics of Health and Fitness

When it comes to health and fitness, it's important to understand the basics. Whether you're a young professional looking to lose weight, reduce stress, or improve your overall health, there are a few key principles that can help you achieve your goals.

First and foremost, it's important to understand that health and fitness are not just about physical appearance. While losing weight or toning your muscles may be a goal, it's important to focus on overall health and wellness. This means taking care of your body through proper nutrition, exercise, and stress management.

One of the most important principles of health and fitness is nutrition. The food you eat plays a major role in your overall health and wellbeing. A balanced diet that includes a variety of fruits, vegetables, lean proteins, and healthy fats is essential for optimal health. If you're looking to lose weight or improve your health, it may be helpful to consult with a nutritionist or registered dietitian to develop a personalized eating plan.

Exercise is another key component of health and fitness. Regular physical activity can improve cardiovascular health, increase strength and flexibility, and reduce stress. Whether you prefer yoga, running, CrossFit, or strength training, finding an activity that you enjoy and can stick to is essential for long-term success.

Stress management is also an important aspect of health and fitness. Chronic stress can have negative effects on both physical and mental health. Mindful meditation, yoga, and other relaxation techniques can help reduce stress and promote overall wellness.

Finally, it's important to remember that health and fitness is a lifelong journey. It's not a quick fix or a one-time event. Making small, sustainable changes to your lifestyle over time can lead to significant improvements in your overall health and wellbeing.

Whether you're just starting out on your health and fitness journey or you're a seasoned pro, it's important to focus on the basics. By prioritizing nutrition, exercise, stress management, and overall wellness, you can achieve your health and fitness goals and live a happier, healthier life.

Setting Realistic Goals for Health and Fitness

One of the biggest reasons why people fail to achieve their health and fitness goals is because they set unrealistic expectations. It's easy to get caught up in the hype of the latest fitness trend or diet fad, but it's important to remember that sustainable change takes time and effort. In this chapter, we'll discuss how to set realistic goals for your health and fitness journey.

1. Identify your why

Before setting any goals, it's important to identify why you want to achieve them. Is it to feel more confident in your body? Improve your overall health? Build strength and endurance? Once you have a clear understanding of your why, you can set specific goals that align with your values and priorities.

2. Be specific

Setting vague goals like "I want to get in shape" or "I want to eat healthier" is unlikely to lead to meaningful change. Instead, be specific about what you want to achieve. For example, "I want to be able to run a 5k without stopping" or "I want to eat 3 servings of vegetables with every meal."

3. Set realistic timelines

It's important to set timelines for your goals, but be sure

they are realistic. If you've never run before, it's unlikely that you'll be able to run a marathon in a month. Set smaller goals along the way, like running a mile without stopping or increasing your distance by 10% each week.

4. Track your progress

Tracking your progress is essential for staying motivated and on track. Keep a journal or use a fitness app to log your workouts, meals, and progress towards your goals. Celebrate your successes along the way and use any setbacks as opportunities to learn and grow.

Remember, health and fitness is a journey, not a destination. By setting realistic goals and staying committed to the process, you can achieve lasting change and live a healthier, more fulfilling life.

Implementing a Sustainable Lifestyle for Health and Fitness

Living a healthy and fit lifestyle is not just about losing weight, it is about building sustainable habits that will help you maintain a healthy body and mind for the long-term. As a young professional, it can be challenging to balance work and other responsibilities with fitness goals. However, with the right mindset and approach, you can achieve your fitness goals while staying productive and focused.

One of the most important aspects of implementing a sustainable lifestyle for health and fitness is developing a routine. Establishing a regular workout schedule and sticking to it will help you build consistency and make exercise a part of your daily routine. Find activities that you enjoy and that fit your schedule, whether it is running, yoga, strength training, or HIIT. Consistency is key to achieving long-term success.

Another important aspect of a sustainable lifestyle is nutrition. Eating a healthy, balanced diet not only helps you maintain a healthy weight but can also improve your mental health, energy levels, and overall well-being. Consider incorporating more plant-based foods into your diet, as they are rich in nutrients and can help reduce your risk of chronic diseases. Additionally, meal prepping can help you save time and stay on track with your nutrition goals.

Stress management is also crucial for maintaining a healthy lifestyle. Yoga and mindful meditation are excellent ways to reduce stress and promote relaxation. CrossFit and strength training can also help you release tension and improve your overall mood. Finding activities that help you manage stress will make it easier to stay consistent with your fitness routine.

Lastly, it is important to listen to your body. Rest and recovery are just as important as exercise, especially as you age. Make sure to get enough sleep and take breaks when needed. Additionally, consider incorporating senior fitness and mobility exercises into your routine to maintain strength and flexibility as you age.

In conclusion, implementing a sustainable lifestyle for health and fitness requires a balance of exercise, nutrition, stress management, and rest and recovery. By developing consistent routines and listening to your body, you can achieve your fitness goals while maintaining productivity and focus as a young professional.

CHAPTER 2: WEIGHT LOSS FOR BUSY PROFESSIONALS

Understanding the Basics of Weight Loss

Weight loss is a common goal for many of us, but it can be difficult to know where to start. In order to lose weight, you need to create a calorie deficit by burning more calories than you consume. This can be achieved through a combination of diet and exercise.

Diet plays a crucial role in weight loss. You need to eat a healthy, balanced diet that is low in calories and high in nutrients. This means focusing on whole foods such as fruits, vegetables, lean proteins, and whole grains, and avoiding processed and high-calorie foods.

Exercise is also important for weight loss. You need to incorporate both cardio and strength training into your routine in order to burn calories and build muscle. Cardio activities such as running, cycling, or swimming can help you burn calories, while strength training activities such as weight lifting or bodyweight exercises can help you build muscle and boost your metabolism.

It's important to remember that weight loss is not a quick fix. It takes time and effort to see results, and it's important to be patient and consistent with your efforts. It's also important to set realistic goals and to focus on making sustainable lifestyle changes rather than quick fixes or fad diets.

In addition to diet and exercise, there are other factors that can impact weight loss. Sleep is crucial for weight loss as it helps regulate hormones that control hunger and metabolism. Stress can also impact weight loss as it can lead to overeating and poor food choices. It's important to prioritize self-care and stress management techniques such as yoga or meditation.

Overall, weight loss is a complex process that involves a combination of diet, exercise, sleep, and stress management. By focusing on making sustainable lifestyle changes and prioritizing your health and wellness, you can achieve your weight loss goals and maintain a healthy and active lifestyle.

Implementing a Sustainable Diet for Weight Loss

Losing weight can be a challenging journey, especially for busy young professionals. With a hectic work schedule and a social life to maintain, finding the time and energy to commit to a healthy lifestyle can be overwhelming.

However, a sustainable diet can be the key to achieving your weight loss goals and improving your overall health and wellbeing. Here are some tips to help you implement a sustainable diet for weight loss:

1. Plan Your Meals

One of the biggest challenges of maintaining a healthy diet is finding the time to cook and prepare your meals. To make things easier, try planning your meals for the week ahead of time. This can help you stay on track and avoid unhealthy food choices when you're busy or stressed.

2. Eat More Whole Foods

Whole foods are nutrient-dense and can help you feel full and satisfied. Try incorporating more fresh fruits and vegetables, lean proteins, and whole grains into your diet. These foods can help you maintain a healthy weight and provide the energy you need to power through your busy day.

3. Limit Processed Foods

Processed foods are often high in calories, sugar, and unhealthy fats. These foods can contribute to weight gain and other health problems. Try to limit your intake of processed foods and opt for whole, nutrient-dense foods instead.

4. Drink More Water

Drinking plenty of water can help you stay hydrated and feel full. Try to drink at least eight glasses of water per day to help you stay on track with your weight loss goals.

5. Practice Mindful Eating

Mindful eating is all about being present and aware of what you're eating. This can help you avoid overeating and make healthier food choices. Try to eat slowly and savor each bite, and pay attention to how your body feels as you eat.

Implementing a sustainable diet for weight loss can be a challenging journey, but it's worth it in the end. By making small changes to your eating habits, you can achieve your weight loss goals and improve your overall health and wellbeing.

Incorporating Exercise into a Busy Schedule

As a young professional, it can be challenging to find time for exercise amidst a busy schedule of work, social events, and other responsibilities. However, incorporating exercise into your routine is crucial for maintaining your physical and mental health. Here are some tips for fitting exercise into even the busiest of schedules:

Prioritize Exercise: Schedule your workout sessions just like you would any other important appointment. Make it a priority to ensure that you don't skip exercise sessions due to other commitments.

Make Use of Short Breaks: Use the short breaks in your workday to squeeze in some exercise. Take a walk around the building, do some stretching exercises or climb a few flights of stairs.

Make It Social: If you find it hard to motivate yourself to exercise, consider joining a fitness class or finding a workout buddy. This way, you can combine exercise with socializing, which can make it more enjoyable and rewarding.

Exercise at Home: If you can't make it to the gym, consider working out at home. There are plenty of online resources and videos that can guide you through at-home workouts without any equipment.

Get Creative: Exercise doesn't have to mean hitting the gym or running on a treadmill. Try other physical activities like dancing, hiking, or swimming. You may be surprised at how much fun you have and how much you can achieve.

Incorporating exercise into a busy schedule takes planning and commitment, but it is possible. By prioritizing exercise and finding creative ways to fit it into your routine, you can improve your overall health and wellbeing. Remember to start small and build up gradually, and most importantly, enjoy the process!

CHAPTER 3: YOGA FOR STRESS RELIEF AND RELAXATION

Understanding the Basics of Yoga

Yoga has been around for thousands of years, but it has only recently gained popularity in the Western world. This ancient practice offers a variety of physical and mental benefits, making it an excellent addition to any fitness routine.

At its core, yoga is a practice that combines physical postures with breathing techniques and meditation. There are many different styles of yoga, each with its own unique approach and focus. Some styles are more intense and physically demanding, while others are gentler and focused on relaxation.

Regardless of the style, yoga is a great way to improve your flexibility, strength, balance, and overall physical fitness.

The postures, or asanas, work to stretch and strengthen different parts of your body, while the breathing techniques help to calm your mind and improve your focus.

One of the most significant benefits of yoga is its ability to reduce stress and promote relaxation. Studies have shown that practicing yoga regularly can lower cortisol levels in the body, which is a hormone associated with stress. This can result in a decrease in anxiety, depression, and overall stress levels.

Yoga is also an excellent way to improve your posture and reduce the risk of injury. By practicing proper alignment and engaging your core muscles, you can strengthen your back, neck, and shoulders, which can help to improve your posture and reduce the risk of injury.

If you are new to yoga, it is essential to start slowly and seek guidance from a qualified instructor. This will help you to learn proper technique and avoid injury. Many yoga studios offer beginner classes, which are a great way to get started.

Overall, yoga is an excellent addition to any fitness routine, offering numerous physical and mental benefits. By practicing regularly, you can improve your flexibility, strength, and balance, while also reducing stress and promoting relaxation. So why not give yoga a try? Your mind and body will thank you.

The Benefits of Yoga for Stress Relief and Relaxation Incorporating Yoga into a Busy Schedule

Yoga is a great way to relieve stress and tension, improve flexibility, and strengthen your body. However, for busy professionals, finding time to practice yoga can be a challenge. Here are some tips for incorporating yoga into your busy schedule:

1. Set a specific time for your yoga practice

One of the best ways to make sure you practice yoga regularly is to schedule it into your day. Whether it's early in the morning or late at night, setting a specific time for your practice can help you stay committed.

2. Find a yoga studio near your workplace

If you work long hours, finding a yoga studio near your workplace can be a great solution. You can attend a class during your lunch break or after work, making it easier to fit yoga into your schedule.

3. Practice yoga at home

If you don't have time to go to a studio, practicing yoga at home can be a great option. There are plenty of online classes and resources available that you can use to create your own practice.

4. Incorporate yoga into your daily routine

You don't have to dedicate a specific time to yoga every day. Instead, try incorporating yoga into your daily routine. For example, you can do a few stretches when you wake up in the morning or before you go to bed at night.

5. Take a yoga retreat

If you're really struggling to find time for yoga, consider taking a yoga retreat. This will allow you to immerse yourself in yoga and completely disconnect from your busy life.

Incorporating yoga into your busy schedule can be a challenge, but it's worth it. By taking the time to practice yoga regularly, you'll improve your physical and mental health, reduce stress, and feel more relaxed and centered in your daily life.

CHAPTER 4: CROSSFIT FOR BEGINNERS

Understanding the Basics of CrossFit

CrossFit is a high-intensity fitness program that has become increasingly popular among fitness enthusiasts. The program is designed to improve overall fitness by incorporating a variety of exercises such as weightlifting, gymnastics, and metabolic conditioning. CrossFit is a great way to challenge yourself physically and mentally, and it can help you achieve your fitness goals.

One of the key components of CrossFit is the use of functional movements. These movements are designed to mimic real-life movements, such as squatting, lifting, and pulling. By focusing on functional movements, CrossFit can help improve overall strength and mobility, which can translate to better performance in everyday life.

Another key component of CrossFit is the use of high-intensity interval training (HIIT). This type of training involves short bursts of intense exercise followed by brief periods of rest. HIIT is an effective way to burn fat and build endurance, making it an ideal training method for those looking to lose weight and improve cardiovascular health.

CrossFit workouts are typically short and intense, lasting anywhere from 10 to 30 minutes. This makes them a great option for busy professionals who may not have a lot of time to devote to exercise. Additionally, CrossFit workouts can be scaled to accommodate any fitness level, making it a great option for beginners and advanced athletes alike.

When starting out with CrossFit, it's important to work with a qualified coach who can guide you through the movements and help you develop proper form. It's also important to listen to your body and take rest days when needed. CrossFit can be intense, so it's important to give your body time to recover.

In conclusion, CrossFit is a great option for those looking to improve their overall fitness. By incorporating functional movements and high-intensity interval training, CrossFit can help you build strength, burn fat, and improve endurance. With the help of a qualified coach, anyone can get started with CrossFit and achieve their fitness goals.

The Benefits of CrossFit for Strength and Endurance

CrossFit is a popular fitness program that has been gaining momentum over the past decade. It is a high-intensity workout that incorporates various movements, including weightlifting, gymnastics, and cardiovascular exercises. CrossFit is designed to improve overall fitness, strength, and endurance. This program is ideal for young professionals who are looking for a fitness routine that is both challenging and rewarding.

One of the biggest benefits of CrossFit is its ability to improve strength. CrossFit workouts incorporate weightlifting movements that target various muscle groups in the body. These movements are performed at high intensity, which helps to build muscle and increase strength. CrossFit also focuses on functional movements that are designed to mimic real-life activities, such as lifting heavy objects or carrying groceries. This type of training helps to improve overall strength, which is essential for young professionals who need to be physically capable of performing their job duties.

Another benefit of CrossFit is its ability to improve endurance. CrossFit workouts typically last 30-60 minutes and are designed to be intense and challenging. These workouts incorporate cardiovascular exercises, such as running, rowing, and cycling, which help to improve cardiovascular endurance. CrossFit also focuses on high-intensity interval training (HIIT), which has been shown to be an effective way to improve endurance and burn fat.

CrossFit is also a great way to improve overall fitness. The program incorporates a variety of movements and exercises, which helps to improve flexibility, agility, and balance. CrossFit workouts are also designed to be scalable, which means they can be modified to suit any fitness level. This makes CrossFit an ideal program for young professionals who are looking to improve their overall fitness and health.

In conclusion, CrossFit is an excellent fitness program for young professionals who are looking to improve their strength, endurance, and overall fitness. This program is challenging, rewarding, and designed to be scalable, making it an ideal choice for individuals of all fitness levels. By incorporating CrossFit into your fitness routine, you can improve your physical capabilities, reduce your risk of injury, and enhance your overall health and well-being.

Incorporating CrossFit into a Busy Schedule

Busy schedules are the norm for young professionals, and finding time to work out can be challenging. However, incorporating CrossFit into your routine can help you stay fit and focused, even with a hectic schedule.

The first step is to find a CrossFit gym that offers classes that fit your schedule. Many CrossFit gyms offer early morning and late evening classes, which can be perfect for those with busy work schedules.

Additionally, some gyms offer lunchtime classes, which can be a great way to fit in a workout during the workday.

Once you've found a gym and class time that works for you, it's important to prioritize your workouts. Make them a non-negotiable part of your schedule, just like any other important appointment. This will help ensure that you stick to your workout routine, even when things get busy.

Another tip for incorporating CrossFit into a busy schedule is to focus on efficiency. CrossFit workouts are designed to be high-intensity and to work multiple muscle groups at once. This means that you can get a great workout in a relatively short amount of time. By focusing on high-intensity, full-body workouts, you can make the most of your limited time.

Finally, it's important to be consistent. Even if you can only make it to the gym a few times a week, make sure to stick to your schedule. Consistency is key when it comes to seeing results and building healthy habits. By staying committed to your CrossFit routine, you'll be able to reap the benefits of improved fitness, increased energy, and reduced stress.

In summary, incorporating CrossFit into a busy schedule requires finding a gym and class time that works for you, prioritizing your workouts, focusing on efficiency, and being consistent. With these tips in mind, you can stay fit and focused, even in the midst of a hectic work schedule.

CHAPTER 5: PALEO DIET FOR ATHLETES

Understanding the Basics of the Paleo Diet

The Paleo diet, also known as the Caveman diet, is a popular dietary plan that focuses on consuming foods that our Paleolithic ancestors would have eaten. The diet consists of whole, unprocessed foods such as lean meats, fish, fruits, vegetables, nuts, and seeds. The Paleo diet excludes processed foods, grains, dairy, and legumes.

The primary goal of the Paleo diet is to improve overall

health and wellness by consuming nutrient-dense, whole foods. While weight loss is a common side effect of the diet, it is not the primary focus.

One of the main benefits of the Paleo diet is its ability to reduce inflammation in the body. By eliminating processed foods and grains that can cause inflammation, the body can heal and recover more efficiently. Additionally, the diet can improve gut health and digestion by removing foods that can irritate the digestive system.

The Paleo diet can be especially beneficial for athletes and active individuals. By consuming whole, nutrient-dense foods, athletes can improve their performance, endurance, and recovery time. The diet can also aid in muscle growth and development by providing the necessary nutrients for optimal recovery and repair.

If you are interested in adopting the Paleo diet, it is important to remember that it is not a one-size-fits-all approach. It is essential to listen to your body and make adjustments as needed. Additionally, it is important to ensure that you are consuming enough calories and nutrients to support your daily activities and fitness routine.

Incorporating the Paleo diet into your lifestyle can be a great way to improve your overall health and wellness. By focusing on whole, unprocessed foods, you can improve your digestion, reduce inflammation, and support your fitness goals.

The Benefits of the Paleo Diet for Athletes

As an athlete, your body requires proper nutrition to perform at its best. The paleo diet can be a great way to fuel your body, improve your performance, and aid in recovery.

The paleo diet focuses on whole, unprocessed foods that our ancestors would have eaten, such as lean meats, vegetables, fruits, nuts, and seeds. It eliminates processed foods, grains, legumes, and dairy, which can often cause inflammation and digestive issues.

One of the benefits of the paleo diet for athletes is improved energy levels. By eliminating processed foods and grains, you can avoid blood sugar spikes and crashes, which can leave you feeling tired and sluggish. Instead, the focus on whole, nutrient-dense foods can provide sustained energy throughout the day.

The paleo diet can also aid in recovery from intense workouts. The diet is high in protein, which is essential for rebuilding muscle tissue after exercise. It also includes healthy fats, which can reduce inflammation and promote healing.

In addition to improved energy levels and recovery, the paleo diet can also aid in weight loss. By eliminating processed foods and grains, you can reduce your overall calorie intake while still feeling satisfied and full. The focus on whole, nutrient-dense foods can also improve your body composition by reducing body fat and increasing lean muscle mass.

It's important to note that the paleo diet may not be appropriate for all athletes. If you have specific dietary needs or restrictions, it's important to consult with a healthcare professional or registered dietitian before making any changes to your diet.

In conclusion, the paleo diet can be a great option for athletes looking to improve their performance, aid in recovery, and maintain a healthy weight. By focusing on whole, unprocessed foods, you can fuel your body with the nutrients it needs to perform at its best.

Incorporating the Paleo Diet into a Busy Schedule

The Paleo diet, also known as the Caveman diet, has become increasingly popular in recent years. It involves eating foods that our ancestors would have eaten in the Paleolithic era, such as lean meats, fish, fruits, vegetables, nuts, and seeds. The idea behind the Paleo diet is that our bodies are better suited to eating these types of foods, and that they can help us maintain a healthy weight, improve our energy levels, and reduce our risk of chronic diseases.

However, for busy professionals, finding the time and energy to prepare Paleo-friendly meals can be a challenge. Here are some tips for incorporating the Paleo diet into a busy schedule:

1. Plan ahead

One of the keys to success with the Paleo diet is planning your meals in advance. This can help you avoid making unhealthy food choices when you're short on time. Take some time each week to plan out your meals and snacks, and make a grocery list of the ingredients you'll need.

2. Prep your meals

Another way to save time when following the Paleo diet is to prep your meals in advance. This could mean cooking large batches of food on the weekends and storing them in the fridge or freezer for later in the week. You could also try meal prepping for the entire week, so you have a variety of healthy meals ready to go when you need them.

3. Keep it simple

When you're short on time, it's important to keep your meals simple. Focus on easy-to-prepare foods like grilled chicken, fish, and vegetables. You can also use a slow cooker or pressure cooker to make meals that require little prep time.

4. Pack your lunch

If you're always on the go, packing your lunch can be a great way to stay on track with the Paleo diet. You can bring along a salad with lean protein, or a wrap made with lettuce instead of bread. This can help you avoid the temptation of fast food or vending machine snacks.

5. Find Paleo-friendly restaurants

When you're eating out, it can be difficult to stick to the Paleo diet. However, many restaurants now offer Paleo-friendly options, so do your research and find places that offer healthy meals that fit within your dietary restrictions.

Incorporating the Paleo diet into a busy schedule can be

challenging, but with a little planning and preparation, it's definitely doable. By focusing on simple, healthy foods and making time to prep your meals, you can enjoy the benefits of the Paleo diet without sacrificing your busy lifestyle.

CHAPTER 6: RUNNING FOR WEIGHT LOSS

Understanding the Basics of Running

Running is one of the most popular forms of exercise and has numerous benefits for your physical and mental health. Whether you are looking to lose weight, improve your cardiovascular fitness, or reduce stress, running can help you achieve your goals. In this subchapter, we will discuss the basics of running and how you can get started on your running journey.

Before you begin running, it is important to have the right equipment. Invest in a good pair of running shoes that provide support and cushioning for your feet. You should also wear comfortable clothing that allows for freedom of movement. Make sure to dress appropriately for the weather, especially if you are running outdoors.

When starting out, it is important to begin slowly and gradually increase your distance and intensity. Start with a brisk walk and gradually add short intervals of running. Over time, you can increase the length of your running intervals and decrease the length of your walking intervals. Aim to run for at least 30 minutes a day, three to four times a week.

As you become more comfortable with running, you can begin to incorporate different types of workouts into your routine. For example, you can include hill sprints, interval training, or long-distance runs. These workouts will help you build endurance, improve your speed, and challenge your body in new ways.

It is also important to pay attention to your form while running. Make sure to keep your shoulders relaxed, your arms bent at a 90-degree angle, and your core engaged. Avoid over striding and land softly on your feet to reduce the impact on your joints.

Lastly, remember to listen to your body and take rest days when needed. If you experience pain or discomfort while running, stop immediately and seek medical attention. Running should be a fun and enjoyable activity that helps you achieve your health and fitness goals.

In conclusion, running is a great way to improve your physical and mental health. By starting slowly, investing in the right equipment, and paying attention to your form, you can develop a running routine that works for you. Incorporate different types of workouts and listen to your body to achieve your running goals.

The Benefits of Running for Weight Loss

Running is a popular form of exercise that can help you shed those extra pounds and achieve your weight loss goals. It is a simple, yet effective way to burn calories, increase your metabolism, and improve your overall health and fitness. Here are some of the benefits of running for weight loss:

1. Burn More Calories

Running is a high-intensity form of exercise that burns more calories than most other forms of exercise. It can help you burn up to 600 calories per hour, depending on your weight, speed, and intensity. This means that running for just 30 minutes a day can help you burn up to 300 calories, which can help you lose weight faster.

2. Boost Your Metabolism

Running can also help boost your metabolism, which is the rate at which your body burns calories. When you run, your body burns more calories even after you stop exercising, which can help you lose weight faster. In fact, studies have shown that running can increase your metabolism by up to 10% for up to 24 hours after you finish your workout.

3. Improve Your Cardiovascular Health

Running is a great way to improve your cardiovascular health, which is important for overall health and fitness. It can help reduce your risk of heart disease, stroke, and other cardiovascular problems. Running can also improve your lung capacity, which can help you breathe more efficiently and feel more energized throughout the day.

4. Reduce Stress and Anxiety

Running can also be a great way to reduce stress and anxiety, which can be a major factor in weight gain. Running releases endorphins, which are natural mood-boosters that can help you feel happier and more relaxed. It can also help you clear your mind and focus on your goals, which can help you stay motivated to achieve your weight loss goals.

5. Improve Your Sleep

Running can also help improve your sleep, which is important for weight loss and overall health and wellness. Running can help you fall asleep faster and stay asleep longer, which can help you wake up feeling more refreshed and energized. This can help you stay focused and motivated throughout the day, which can help you achieve your weight loss goals faster

In conclusion, running is a great way to lose weight, improve your health and fitness, reduce stress and anxiety, and improve your sleep. If you're a young professional looking to lose weight and improve your overall health and wellness, running is a great place to start. Just remember to start slowly and gradually increase your speed and distance over time to avoid injury and burnout.

Incorporating Running into a Busy Schedule

Running is a great way to improve your fitness and lose weight, but it can be challenging to fit it into a busy schedule. However, with a little planning and dedication, you can make running a regular part of your routine.

First, consider your schedule and find pockets of time that you can dedicate to running. This may mean waking up earlier in the morning or skipping lunch to fit in a quick run. You can also try running during your commute by running to work or home. This can help you save time and stay active during your daily routine.

Another way to incorporate running into your busy schedule is to make it a social activity. Find a running buddy or join a running group to make your runs more enjoyable and social. This can help you stay motivated and accountable, and it can also help you meet new people who share your fitness goals.

If you're new to running, start slow and gradually increase your distance and speed. This can help you avoid injury and build up your endurance. You can also try mixing up your running routine by adding in intervals or hills to keep things interesting.

Finally, make sure you have the right gear and equipment to support your running routine. This may include comfortable running shoes, moisture-wicking clothing, and a hydration pack or belt. Investing in quality gear can help you stay comfortable and safe during your runs, and it can also help you stay motivated to keep running.

Incorporating running into a busy schedule may seem challenging, but with a little planning and dedication, it can be done. Whether you're a beginner or an experienced runner, make running a regular part of your routine to improve your fitness, lose weight, and stay healthy.

CHAPTER 7: SENIOR FITNESS AND MOBILITY

Understanding the Basics of Senior Fitness

As we age, it becomes increasingly important to prioritize our health and fitness. Senior fitness is all about staying active and maintaining mobility, balance, and strength. In this section, we'll dive into the basics of senior fitness, including why it's important, what types of exercises are best, and how to stay motivated.

Why is Senior Fitness Important?

As we age, our bodies naturally undergo changes that can impact our ability to move and perform everyday activities. However, staying active and maintaining a regular exercise routine can help to counteract these changes and promote overall health and wellness.

Regular exercise can help to:

- Improve bone density and muscle strength
- Maintain balance and coordination
- Reduce the risk of falls and injuries
- Boost cardiovascular health
- Improve cognitive function and mental health
- Enhance overall quality of life

What Types of Exercises are Best?

When it comes to senior fitness, it's important to focus on exercises that will help to maintain mobility, balance, and strength. Some of the best types of exercises for seniors include:

- **Aerobic exercise:** This includes activities like walking, swimming, and cycling, which can help to improve cardiovascular health and endurance.

- **Strength training:** This involves using weights, resistance bands, or bodyweight exercises to build and maintain muscle strength.

- **Balance exercises:** These exercises can help to reduce the risk of falls and improve overall balance and coordination.

- **Flexibility exercises:** Stretching and range-of-motion exercises can help to maintain mobility and reduce stiffness.

How to Stay Motivated with Senior Fitness

Staying motivated with senior fitness can be challenging, but there are a few strategies that can help:

- **Set realistic goals:** Start with small, achievable goals and gradually increase the intensity and duration of your workouts.

- **Find a workout buddy:** Working out with a friend or family member can make exercise more enjoyable and keep you accountable.

- **Mix it up:** Try different types of exercises and workouts to keep things interesting and prevent boredom.

- Celebrate your progress: Take time to acknowledge and celebrate your accomplishments, no matter how small they may seem.

Overall, senior fitness is an essential component of overall health and wellness. By staying active and focusing on exercises that promote mobility, balance, and strength, you can maintain your independence and enjoy a high quality of life as you age.

The Benefits of Senior Fitness for Mobility and Independence

As we age, we tend to experience a decline in our physical abilities, which can lead to a loss of independence. However, regular exercise and physical activity can help seniors maintain their mobility and independence for longer.

One of the main benefits of senior fitness is improved balance and coordination. Falls are a major concern for older adults, and by improving their balance and coordination, seniors can reduce their risk of falls and related injuries. Strength training exercises, such as squats and lunges, can help improve balance and stability.

Regular exercise can also help seniors maintain their strength and flexibility. As we age, our muscles and joints become stiffer, which can make it difficult to perform everyday tasks. However, by incorporating stretching and resistance training exercises into their routine, seniors can improve their flexibility and muscle strength, making it easier to perform tasks such as getting up from a chair or carrying groceries.

In addition to the physical benefits, senior fitness can also have a positive impact on mental health. Exercise has been shown to reduce symptoms of depression and anxiety, and can improve cognitive function and memory. For seniors, this can mean better overall mental health and a greater sense of independence and self-confidence.

Finally, senior fitness can also have social benefits. Group fitness classes and activities can provide seniors with opportunities to socialize and connect with others who share similar interests. This can be especially important for seniors who may be isolated or lonely.

In conclusion, senior fitness is essential for maintaining mobility and independence in older adults. By incorporating regular exercise and physical activity into their routine, seniors can improve their balance, strength, flexibility, and mental health, while also enjoying the social benefits of group fitness activities.

Incorporating Senior Fitness into a Busy Schedule

As young professionals, our schedules can get pretty hectic. Between work, family commitments, and social events, it can be challenging to find time for fitness. However, it's essential to prioritize exercise, especially as we age. Incorporating senior fitness into your busy schedule doesn't have to be a daunting task. There are several ways to stay active and healthy, even with a jam-packed calendar.

Firstly, it's essential to make fitness a priority. Schedule your workouts like you would any other appointment. Set aside specific times each week to exercise, and stick to them. Whether it's before work, during lunch, or after dinner, find a time that works best for you and make it a habit.

Secondly, consider joining a gym or fitness class. Having a set time and place to work out can help keep you accountable. Plus, working out in a group can be motivating and fun. Many gyms and fitness studios offer senior fitness classes that cater to older adults' needs. These classes typically focus on low-impact exercises that improve mobility, balance, and strength.

Thirdly, find ways to incorporate exercise into your daily routine. If you have a desk job, take breaks every hour to stretch and move around. Take the stairs instead of the elevator, and park farther away from the entrance to get extra steps in. Even small changes can make a big difference in your overall health and fitness levels.

Lastly, make sure you're incorporating a variety of exercises into your routine. As we age, it's important to focus on improving mobility, balance, and strength. Incorporating yoga or Pilates into your routine can help improve flexibility and balance. Strength training can help maintain muscle mass and improve bone density. And cardio, such as walking or cycling, can improve cardiovascular health and aid in weight loss.

In conclusion, incorporating senior fitness into a busy schedule is possible with a little planning and dedication. Making fitness a priority, joining a gym or fitness class, finding ways to incorporate exercise into your daily routine, and varying your workouts are all excellent strategies for staying active and healthy as you age. Remember, it's never too late to start prioritizing your health and fitness.

CHAPTER 8: PLANT-BASED NUTRITION FOR IMPROVED HEALTH

Understanding the Basics of Plant-Based Nutrition

The plant-based diet has gained popularity in recent years, and for good reason. It has been linked to lower risk of chronic diseases such as heart disease, diabetes, and cancer, as well as weight loss and improved overall health. If you are a young professional looking to improve your health and fitness, incorporating more plant-based foods into your diet can be a great step in the right direction.

What is a Plant-Based Diet?

A plant-based diet is centered around foods derived from plants, such as fruits, vegetables, whole grains, legumes, nuts, and seeds. It may or may not include small amounts of animal products, depending on your personal preference and beliefs. The focus is on whole, minimally processed foods that are nutrient-dense and high in fiber.

Benefits of a Plant-Based Diet

A plant-based diet has numerous health benefits, including:

1. Lower risk of chronic diseases: Studies have shown that a plant-based diet can lower your risk of chronic diseases, such as heart disease, diabetes, and cancer.

2. Weight loss: Plant-based diets are typically lower in calories and higher in fiber, which can lead to weight loss.

3. Improved digestion: The high fiber content in plant-based foods can improve digestion and prevent constipation.

4. Better skin: Plant-based foods are rich in antioxidants, which can improve skin health and reduce the signs of aging.

5. Increased energy: The high nutrient content in plant-based foods can increase energy levels and reduce fatigue.

How to Incorporate More Plant-Based Foods into Your Diet

If you are looking to incorporate more plant-based foods into your diet, here are some tips:

1. Start small: Begin by adding one plant-based meal or snack per day, and gradually increase as you become more comfortable with the diet.

2. Experiment with new foods: Try new fruits, vegetables, whole grains, legumes, nuts, and seeds to keep your diet interesting and varied.

3. Plan your meals: Make a meal plan for the week to ensure that you have enough plant-based options available.

4. Get creative: Look up plant-based recipes online, and experiment with new flavors and cooking techniques.

5. Be mindful of your nutritional needs: Make sure that you are getting enough protein, iron, calcium, and other essential nutrients in your diet.

In conclusion, a plant-based diet can be a great way to improve your health and fitness as a young professional. By incorporating more plant-based foods into your diet, you can lower your risk of chronic diseases, lose weight, improve digestion, and increase your energy levels. Remember to start small, experiment with new foods, plan your meals, get creative, and be mindful of your nutritional needs.

The Benefits of Plant-Based Nutrition for Improved Health

Plant-based nutrition has been gaining popularity in recent years, and for good reason. This type of diet is based on whole, unprocessed foods that come from plants. It includes fruits, vegetables, legumes, grains, nuts, and seeds. By eliminating animal products, this diet is naturally low in saturated fat and cholesterol, making it a great option for those looking to improve their health.

One of the main benefits of plant-based nutrition is improved heart health. Studies have shown that a diet rich in fruits, vegetables, and whole grains can lower blood pressure and reduce the risk of heart disease. Additionally, a plant-based diet can help lower cholesterol levels, which is a major risk factor for heart disease.

Plant-based nutrition can also help with weight management. Since this type of diet is naturally lower in calories, it can help with weight loss and weight maintenance. In fact, studies have shown that those who follow a plant-based diet tend to have a lower body mass index (BMI) compared to those who consume animal products.

Another benefit of plant-based nutrition is improved digestion. The high fiber content in plant-based foods can help prevent constipation and promote regular bowel movements. Additionally, the natural enzymes in fruits and vegetables can help with digestion and nutrient absorption.

Plant-based nutrition can also improve overall energy levels and mental clarity. Since this type of diet is rich in vitamins and minerals, it can help provide the body with the nutrients it needs to function properly.

Additionally, plant-based foods are often easier to digest, which can help prevent feelings of fatigue and sluggishness.

In conclusion, plant-based nutrition offers numerous benefits for improved health. From improved heart health to weight management and improved digestion, this type of diet is a great option for those looking to improve their overall health and well-being. Whether you're a young professional looking to improve your health or an athlete looking to fuel your body for optimal performance, plant-based nutrition is a great choice.

Incorporating Plant-Based Nutrition into a Busy Schedule

As young professionals, it can be challenging to maintain a healthy diet while juggling work, social life, and other responsibilities. However, incorporating plant-based nutrition into your busy schedule can provide numerous health benefits and help you stay on track with your fitness goals. Here are some tips to help you incorporate plant-based nutrition into your busy lifestyle:

1. Plan your meals ahead of time:

Planning your meals ahead of time can save you time and ensure that you have healthy meal options available. Take some time on the weekends to plan your meals for the week, and make a grocery list of the ingredients you'll need. This will help you avoid impulse purchases and ensure that you have healthy food options available, even when you're short on time.

2. Batch cook your meals:

Batch cooking can save you time and ensure that you have healthy meals available throughout the week. Choose a day to prepare your meals for the week and store them in the refrigerator or freezer. This will help you avoid unhealthy fast food options when you're short on time.

3. Keep healthy snacks on hand:

Keeping healthy snacks on hand can help you avoid

unhealthy snacking habits. Stock up on fresh fruits, vegetables, nuts, and seeds, and keep them in your office, car, or bag. This will help you stay full and energized throughout the day.

4. Try new plant-based recipes:

Trying new plant-based recipes can help you stay motivated and interested in your diet. Look for new recipes online or in cookbooks, and experiment with different ingredients and flavors. This will help you discover new plant-based foods that you enjoy and keep your diet interesting.

5. Incorporate plant-based protein sources:

Incorporating plant-based protein sources into your diet can help you meet your nutritional needs and support your fitness goals. Some examples of plant-based protein sources include tofu, tempeh, lentils, chickpeas, and quinoa. Try incorporating these foods into your meals to add flavor and nutritional value.

In conclusion, incorporating plant-based nutrition into a busy schedule can be challenging, but it's possible with some planning and dedication. By planning your meals ahead of time, batch cooking, keeping healthy snacks on hand, trying new plant-based recipes, and incorporating plant-based protein sources, you can improve your health.

CHAPTER 9: HIGH-INTENSITY INTERVAL TRAINING (HIIT) FOR FAT LOSS

Understanding the Basics of HIIT

High-intensity interval training (HIIT) is a popular fitness trend that has gained a lot of attention in recent years. It is a form of exercise that involves short bursts of intense activity followed by periods of rest or lower intensity exercise. HIIT workouts can be done in as little as 20 minutes, making them a great option for busy professionals who want to get fit but don't have a lot of time to spare.

The benefits of HIIT are numerous. Research has shown that HIIT can help improve cardiovascular fitness, increase metabolism, reduce body fat, and improve insulin sensitivity. It can also help build muscle and improve athletic performance. HIIT is a great way to challenge yourself and push your limits, and it can be a fun and exciting way to get in shape.

To get started with HIIT, it is important to understand the basics. First, you need to choose an activity that you enjoy and that challenges you. This could be running, cycling, swimming, or any other form of cardio exercise. Next, you need to set up a routine that includes short bursts of intense activity followed by periods of rest or lower intensity exercise.

For example, you could do 30 seconds of sprinting followed by 30 seconds of walking or jogging, and repeat this cycle for 20 minutes.

It is important to warm up and cool down properly before and after your HIIT workout. This will help prevent injuries and ensure that your body is ready for the intense activity. You should also make sure that you are properly hydrated and fueled before your workout to ensure that you have the energy to complete it.

As with any form of exercise, it is important to listen to your body and adjust your routine as needed. If you are new to HIIT, start with shorter workouts and gradually increase the intensity and duration as you become more comfortable. It is also important to rest and recover between workouts to allow your body to heal and rebuild.

In summary, HIIT is a great option for busy professionals who want to get fit and healthy. By understanding the basics and incorporating HIIT into your routine, you can improve your health, increase your fitness, and achieve your weight loss goals.

The Benefits of HIIT for Fat Loss and Endurance

High-intensity interval training (HIIT) is a type of workout that has been gaining popularity in recent years. It involves short bursts of intense exercise followed by periods of rest or low-intensity exercise. HIIT has been shown to be an effective method for both fat loss and endurance training. In this subchapter, we will discuss the benefits of HIIT for fat loss and endurance and why it is an excellent choice for busy young professionals.

One of the primary benefits of HIIT is that it can help you burn more calories in a shorter amount of time. Studies have shown that HIIT can burn up to 30% more calories than traditional cardio workouts. This means that you can get a more effective workout in less time. For busy young professionals who are short on time, HIIT can be a lifesaver.

Another benefit of HIIT is that it can help you lose fat while preserving muscle mass. Traditional cardio workouts can cause you to lose muscle mass along with fat. However, HIIT has been shown to preserve muscle mass while still helping you lose fat. This is important because muscle mass is important for maintaining a healthy metabolism and overall health.

HIIT can also improve your endurance. Because HIIT involves short bursts of intense exercise followed by rest, it can help increase your anaerobic threshold. This means that you will be able to perform high-intensity exercise for longer periods of time without getting tired. This can be particularly useful for athletes who need to perform at high levels for extended periods of time.

Finally, HIIT can be a fun and varied way to exercise. There are many different types of HIIT workouts, so you can mix things up and keep your workouts interesting. This can help prevent boredom and keep you motivated to exercise regularly.

In conclusion, if you are a busy young professional looking to lose fat and improve your endurance, HIIT is an excellent choice. It can help you burn more calories, preserve muscle mass, improve your endurance, and keep your workouts interesting. Incorporating HIIT into your fitness routine can help you achieve your goals and maintain a healthy lifestyle.

Incorporating HIIT into a Busy Schedule

High-Intensity Interval Training (HIIT) is an effective way to lose weight, increase endurance, and improve overall fitness. However, with a busy schedule, finding the time to fit in a full HIIT workout might seem daunting. But, with the right approach, it's possible to incorporate HIIT into your busy schedule and get the benefits of this workout.

The first step is to choose the right HIIT workout. There are many HIIT workouts available, but not all are suitable for those with a busy schedule. Look for workouts that are short and can be done in a small space. For example, a 20-minute HIIT workout that involves bodyweight exercises like squats, lunges, and push-ups can be easily done in a living room.

Another way to incorporate HIIT into a busy schedule is to break up the workout into smaller segments. Instead of doing a 20-minute workout in one go, you can do two 10-minute HIIT workouts, one in the morning and one in the evening. This approach is especially useful for those who don't have a lot of time in the morning or evening but can spare a few minutes during the day.

If you're someone who has a tight schedule throughout the day, you can try incorporating HIIT into your daily routine. For example, you can do a quick HIIT session during your lunch break or in between meetings.

This approach not only saves time but also helps in breaking up the monotony of a busy workday.

Lastly, if you're someone who travels frequently, you can take advantage of HIIT workouts that don't require any equipment. These workouts can be done in a hotel room or any other small space. All you need is a bit of motivation and the willingness to sweat it out.

In conclusion, incorporating HIIT into a busy schedule is not only doable, but also beneficial for your health and fitness. By choosing the right workout, breaking it up into smaller segments, incorporating it into your daily routine, or taking advantage of travel-friendly workouts, you can fit HIIT into your busy lifestyle and reap the rewards of this high-intensity workout.

CHAPTER 10: STRENGTH TRAINING FOR WOMEN

Understanding the Basics of Strength Training

Strength training is a great way to improve your overall health and fitness. It is a type of exercise that involves lifting weights or using resistance to build muscle strength and endurance. This type of training is beneficial for both men and women, and it can help you achieve your fitness goals faster and more effectively.

The Benefits of Strength Training

Strength training offers many benefits, including:

1. Increased muscle strength and endurance

2. Improved muscle tone and definition

3. Increased bone density

4. Improved balance and coordination

5. Increased metabolism

6. Reduced risk of injury

7. Improved mental health and well-being

8. Enhanced athletic performance

The Basics of Strength Training

Strength training involves using weights or resistance to challenge your muscles. The resistance can come from free weights, weight machines, resistance bands, or even your own body weight. The goal is to work your muscles to fatigue, which means you can no longer perform another repetition with good form.

To get started with strength training, you should first determine your goals. Do you want to build muscle, increase endurance, or improve your overall fitness? Once you know your goals, you can design a strength training program that will help you achieve them.

Your strength training program should include exercises for all the major muscle groups, including the chest, back, shoulders, arms, legs, and abs. It is important to vary your exercises and increase the weight or resistance as you get stronger.

Tips for Success

To get the most out of your strength training program, follow these tips:

1. Start with light weights and gradually increase the weight as you get stronger.

2. Use proper form and technique to avoid injury.

3. Allow your muscles to rest for at least 48 hours between workouts.

4. Incorporate cardio and stretching into your fitness routine for overall health and fitness.

5. Consider working with a personal trainer to design a customized strength training program that meets your needs and goals.

In conclusion, strength training is an effective way to improve your overall health and fitness. By incorporating strength training into your fitness routine, you can achieve your goals faster and more effectively. Start with the basics and gradually increase your weight and resistance to build muscle strength and endurance. With a little patience and dedication, you can achieve your fitness goals and improve your overall well-being.

The Benefits of Strength Training for Women's Health

Strength training has been long associated with men, but it

is a highly effective and beneficial exercise for women as well. Women who engage in strength training can enjoy a multitude of benefits for their overall health and well-being. Here are some of the benefits of strength training for women's health.

Improved Bone Density

As women age, they are at a higher risk of developing osteoporosis, a condition that weakens bones and makes them more prone to fractures. Strength training is an effective way to increase bone density and reduce the risk of osteoporosis. Weight-bearing exercises like squats, lunges, and deadlifts can help build stronger bones, especially in the hips and spine.

Increased Muscle Mass

Strength training helps women build lean muscle mass, which can help improve their overall body composition. Having more muscle mass can also help boost metabolism, making it easier for women to maintain a healthy weight.

Reduced Risk of Chronic Diseases

Strength training has been shown to lower the risk of chronic diseases like type 2 diabetes, heart disease, and certain types of cancer. It can also improve insulin sensitivity and help regulate blood sugar levels.

Improved Mental Health

Strength training has numerous benefits for mental health. It can help reduce anxiety and depression, improve mood, and boost self-confidence. It can also help improve cognitive function and memory.

Better Posture and Balance

Strength training can help improve posture and balance, which can reduce the risk of falls and injuries, especially in older women. Exercises like planks, push-ups, and squats can help strengthen core muscles and improve overall stability.

In conclusion, strength training is a highly effective exercise that offers numerous benefits for women's health. It can improve bone density, increase muscle mass, reduce the risk of chronic diseases, and improve mental health, posture, and balance. Incorporating strength training into a fitness routine can help women achieve their health and fitness goals and lead a healthy and fulfilling life.

Incorporating Strength Training into a Busy Schedule

Strength training is an essential component of a well-rounded fitness program. It helps improve bone density, increase muscle mass, and boost metabolism. It also enhances overall physical performance, reduces the risk of injury, and helps prevent chronic diseases.

But with a busy schedule, finding the time to strength train can be challenging. Here are some tips to help you incorporate strength training into your busy life.

1. Schedule Your Workout

The first step to incorporating strength training into your schedule is to make it a priority. Plan your workout at a time that works best for you, and stick to it. Whether it's before work, during lunch break, or after work, choose a time that works best for your schedule and make it a habit.

2. Choose Efficient Workouts

When you have limited time, choosing efficient workouts is key. High-intensity interval training (HIIT) and circuit training are great options as they provide a full-body workout in a short amount of time. These workouts can be completed in as little as 20 minutes and are great for burning fat and building muscle.

3. Make Use of Your Environment

You don't need a gym or fancy equipment to strength train. Use your environment to your advantage. Bodyweight exercises such as push-ups, squats, and lunges can be done anywhere. You can also use household items such as water bottles or backpacks filled with books as weights.

4. Incorporate Strength Training into Your Daily Routine

Incorporating strength training into your daily routine can help you stay consistent. Take the stairs instead of the elevator, do calf raises while brushing your teeth, or do lunges while waiting for the bus. These small changes can add up and help you reach your fitness goals.

5. Find a Workout Partner

Having a workout partner can help keep you accountable and motivated. Find a friend or coworker who shares your fitness goals and schedule workouts together. You can also join a fitness class or group to meet like-minded individuals.

Incorporating strength training into a busy schedule may seem daunting, but with these tips, it can be done. By making it a priority, choosing efficient workouts, using your environment, incorporating it into your daily routine, and finding a workout partner, you can achieve your fitness goals and improve your overall health and well-being.

CHAPTER 11: MINDFUL MEDITATION FOR MENTAL AND PHYSICAL WELLNESS

Understanding the Basics of Mindful Meditation

Mindful meditation is a practice that has been around for centuries and has been gaining popularity in recent years. This technique involves training your mind to focus on the present moment and is an effective way to reduce stress, anxiety, and improve overall mental and physical wellness. If you are a young professional looking to improve your health and fitness, incorporating mindful meditation into your routine is a great way to start.

To begin with, it is essential to understand the basics of mindful meditation. The first step is to find a quiet and comfortable place to sit or lie down. Next, close your eyes and focus on your breath. Notice how your body feels as you inhale and exhale. If your mind starts to wander, gently bring your focus back to your breath. It is normal for your mind to wander during meditation, so do not get discouraged if this happens. The key is to be patient and persistent.

Another important aspect of mindful meditation is to be non-judgmental. Rather than criticizing yourself for not being able to focus, acknowledge your thoughts and let them go. The goal is not to eliminate all thoughts but to observe them without judgment.

One of the benefits of mindful meditation is its ability to reduce stress and anxiety. By focusing on your breath and being present in the moment, you can calm your mind and reduce the negative effects of stress on your body. Regular practice of mindful meditation has been shown to improve overall mental health and reduce symptoms of depression and anxiety.

In addition to mental health benefits, mindful meditation has been shown to improve physical health as well. By reducing stress and anxiety, you may notice improvements in your sleep quality and immune function. It can also be a useful tool for managing chronic pain and improving cardiovascular health.

In conclusion, mindful meditation is a simple yet powerful way to improve your mental and physical wellness. Incorporating this practice into your daily routine can have a significant impact on your health and fitness. Whether you are a beginner or have been practicing for a while, remember to be patient, non-judgmental, and persistent in your efforts.

The Benefits of Mindful Meditation for Mental and Physical Wellness

As young professionals, the demands of our daily lives can take a toll on our mental and physical health. With long working hours, tight deadlines, and social obligations, it can be challenging to find time to prioritize our well-being. However, incorporating mindful meditation into our daily routine can provide numerous benefits for our mental and physical wellness.

Mindful meditation involves focusing your attention on the present moment, being aware of your thoughts and feelings without judgment. Practicing mindfulness can help reduce stress, anxiety, and depression, which are common mental health issues faced by young professionals. Through regular meditation, you can learn to manage your emotions better and develop a sense of calmness, which can improve your overall well-being.

In addition to mental health benefits, mindful meditation can also have positive effects on your physical health. Studies have shown that mindfulness can lower blood pressure, improve sleep quality, and boost immunity, among other benefits. Incorporating mindful meditation into your fitness routine can also enhance your performance and prevent injuries by improving your focus, posture, and body awareness.

Implementing mindful meditation into your daily routine does not have to be time-consuming or complicated. Start with a few minutes each day and gradually increase the duration as you become more comfortable with the practice. You can meditate anywhere, whether it's in a quiet room, during your commute, or even while walking. There are also many resources available, including apps, videos, and classes, to help you get started and stay motivated.

Incorporating mindful meditation into your daily routine can provide numerous benefits for your mental and physical wellness. By taking the time to focus on yourself and your well-being, you can improve your overall quality of life and become more fit and focused in all aspects of your life.

Incorporating Mindful Meditation into a Busy Schedule

In today's fast-paced world, it can be difficult to find time to take care of ourselves. Between work, family, and other obligations, it's easy to feel overwhelmed and stressed out. But taking care of our mental and physical health is crucial for leading a fulfilling life. That's where mindful meditation comes in.

Mindful meditation is a practice that involves focusing your attention on the present moment. It can help reduce stress, anxiety, and depression, and improve overall mental and physical wellness. But how can you incorporate mindful meditation into a busy schedule?

First, start small. You don't need to meditate for hours on end to see the benefits. Even just five minutes a day can make a difference. Set aside a specific time each day to meditate, whether it's first thing in the morning or before bed.

Second, find a quiet and comfortable space to meditate. It could be a corner of your bedroom, a park bench, or even your office. Make sure you won't be disturbed during your meditation practice.

Next, choose a meditation style that works for you. There are many different types of meditation, from guided meditations to mindfulness exercises. Experiment with different styles to find one that resonates with you.

Finally, be patient with yourself. Meditation is a skill that takes time and practice to develop. It's normal to have thoughts and distractions during your practice. Instead of getting frustrated, simply acknowledge them and refocus your attention on your breath or your chosen meditation technique.

Incorporating mindful meditation into your busy schedule may seem daunting at first, but it's worth the effort. Start small, find a quiet space, choose a meditation style that works for you, and be patient with yourself. With practice, you'll soon reap the benefits of this powerful practice.

CONCLUSION

The Importance of Health and Fitness for Young Professionals

As a young professional, you may find yourself constantly juggling work, personal life, and social obligations. With so much on your plate, it can be easy to neglect your health and fitness. However, prioritizing your physical and mental well-being is crucial to maintaining a successful and fulfilling career.

First and foremost, taking care of your health can improve your productivity and focus at work. Exercise releases endorphins, which can boost your mood and energy levels. This can lead to better concentration, creativity, and problem-solving skills. Additionally, a healthy diet can provide the nutrients your brain needs to function at its best.

Incorporating fitness into your routine can also help manage stress. Yoga, for example, is a great way to relieve tension and promote relaxation. It can improve your flexibility and balance, as well as reduce anxiety and depression. CrossFit, on the other hand, offers a high-intensity workout that can challenge you both mentally and physically.

If weight loss is a goal for you, running can be an effective way to shed pounds. It's a low-cost activity that can be done anywhere, and it burns a significant number of calories. High-intensity interval training (HIIT) is another option for fat loss, as it involves short bursts of intense exercise followed by periods of rest.

Strength training is also important, particularly for women. It can increase muscle mass and bone density, leading to a stronger and more resilient body. Plus, it can help prevent injuries and improve posture.

Of course, nutrition is a crucial component of overall health and fitness. A plant-based diet can provide the vitamins, minerals, and antioxidants your body needs to function optimally. The paleo diet, which emphasizes whole foods and eliminates processed items, may also be beneficial for athletes and those looking to lose weight.

Finally, it's important to practice self-care for your mental health. Mindful meditation can help you manage stress and improve your emotional well-being. It involves focusing your attention on the present moment, without judgment or distraction.

In summary, prioritizing your health and fitness as a young

professional can lead to improved productivity, reduced stress, and a better quality of life. Whether you prefer yoga, running, or strength training, finding a fitness routine that works for you is essential. Additionally, nourishing your body with whole, nutrient-dense foods can help you reach your health goals. By making these habits a priority, you can set yourself up for success in both your personal and professional life.

The Benefits of a Sustainable Lifestyle for Health and Fitness

Living a sustainable lifestyle has numerous benefits for both your health and fitness. It is not only good for the environment, but it can also help you achieve your health and fitness goals. Here are some of the benefits of a sustainable lifestyle for your health and fitness:

1. Helps you maintain a healthy weight.

A sustainable lifestyle involves making healthier food choices and incorporating more physical activity into your daily routine. This can help you maintain a healthy weight and reduce the risk of obesity-related diseases such as diabetes and heart disease.

2. Boosts your energy levels.

Eating a balanced diet and engaging in regular physical activity can help boost your energy levels, making you more productive and focused throughout the day.

3. Improves your mental health.

Living a sustainable lifestyle can also have a positive impact on your mental health. Engaging in physical activity and consuming a healthy diet can help reduce stress and anxiety, and improve your overall mood.

4. Reduces the risk of chronic diseases.

A sustainable lifestyle involves consuming more whole foods and less processed foods, which can help reduce the risk of chronic diseases such as cancer, heart disease, and diabetes.

5. Enhances your athletic performance.

For athletes, a sustainable lifestyle can help enhance their athletic performance. Consuming a diet rich in whole foods can provide the necessary nutrients for optimal performance, while engaging in regular physical activity can help improve strength, endurance, and speed.

6. Improves your overall quality of life.

Living a sustainable lifestyle can help improve your overall quality of life. By making healthier choices and engaging in physical activity, you can enjoy a longer, healthier, and more fulfilling life.

In conclusion, adopting a sustainable lifestyle can have numerous benefits for your health and fitness. By making healthier choices and incorporating more physical activity into your daily routine, you can achieve your health and fitness goals while also helping to protect the environment. So why not start living sustainably today?

The Future of Health and Fitness for Young Professionals.

As young professionals, our busy schedules often leave little time for prioritizing our health and fitness. However, the future of health and fitness for young professionals is looking bright, with new innovations and trends emerging that make it easier than ever to maintain a healthy lifestyle.

One of the most exciting trends in health and fitness is the rise of wearable technology. Devices like fitness trackers and smartwatches allow us to track our physical activity, monitor our heart rate, and even analyze our sleep patterns. With this data at our fingertips, we can make more informed decisions about our health and fitness goals, and stay motivated as we work towards achieving them.

Another trend that is gaining popularity is the use of virtual fitness classes. With the rise of streaming services like Peloton and Beachbody, we can now access high-quality fitness classes from the comfort of our own homes. This is particularly beneficial for busy professionals who may not have the time to attend a gym or fitness studio.

In addition to these technological advancements, there are also new and innovative approaches to nutrition that are emerging. For example, the plant-based nutrition movement is gaining traction, with more and more people turning to a vegetarian or vegan diet for improved health and wellness.

These trends are all geared towards making it easier for

young professionals to prioritize their health and fitness, even when their schedules are packed. By leveraging technology, virtual fitness classes, and new approaches to nutrition, we can stay fit and focused, no matter how busy our lives may be.

Of course, it's important to remember that there is no one-size-fits-all approach to health and fitness. Each of us is unique, with different goals, preferences, and lifestyles. It's important to take the time to find what works best for us, whether that be yoga for stress relief, CrossFit for beginners, or running for weight loss.

Ultimately, the future of health and fitness for young professionals is bright, with new innovations and trends emerging every day. By staying informed and open to new approaches, we can maintain a healthy and balanced lifestyle, even amidst the demands of our busy professional lives.

ABOUT THE AUTHOR

Sales and Marketing Professional with more than 25 Plus years of diversified experience for both transnational and national pharmaceutical companies such as Merck & Co. Inc. NV Organon, AkzoNobel, and OBS Pakistan (Pvt.) Limited. Moreover, he is a university Professor and has more than 10 years' experience of teaching, research and supervising dissertations for MBA, MS. M.Phil., and Ph.D. level students. He is an author and coauthor of more than 200 publications, in which he has written more than 80 impact factor research articles, and 20 books.